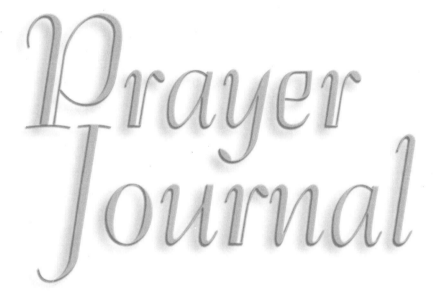

Prayer Journal

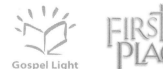

Gospel Light

FIRST PLACE

Gospel Light is an evangelical Christian publisher dedicated to serving the local church. We believe God's vision for Gospel Light is to provide church leaders with biblical, user-friendly materials that will help them evangelize, disciple and minister to children, youth and families.

It is our prayer that this Gospel Light resource will help you discover biblical truth for your own life and help you minister to others. May God richly bless you.

For a free catalog of resources from Gospel Light, please contact your Christian supplier or contact us at 1-800-4-GOSPEL or www.gospellight.com.

William T. Greig, Publisher
Kyle Duncan, Associate Publisher
Pam Weston, Editor
Samantha A. Hsu, Designer, Cover Designer

THE VALUE OF PRAYER JOURNALS

A PERSONAL TESTIMONY

Believing that God wants His children to pray, I began writing my prayers in April 1990. For several years, I had resisted praying in this manner. Being a fun-loving individual, I felt that writing my prayers would be time consuming, to say the least. At that time, my prayer life was not something I found pleasant or rewarding. I felt five minutes was a long time to pray. My thoughts would begin to wander and before I knew it, I was planning the day ahead, rather than praying. I had attended seminars on prayer for years. I thought some secret formula must exist that would make me a mighty prayer warrior. That is until I began prayer journaling.

The greatest benefit I have received from writing my prayers is the total focus on praying while I am writing. My mind is focused because it is difficult to write and think of other things at the same time. Also, the Holy Spirit directs my praying when my mind is tuned in to God. My faith grows tremendously as I go back through my journal and highlight the many answers to prayer in my life.

God has taught me many truths through journaling. I have learned to praise Him in all things. Trials in my life may seem like roadblocks to me, but God sees these trials as stepping-stones to victory and spiritual growth. Journaling has taught me that God hears and answers all my prayers. When I pray within the framework of God's will, His answer is always a resounding yes! When God tells me no, He does so because I have asked something contrary to His will for my life. Many times what I perceive as His "No" is only "Wait, my child—the timing is not yet right."

Another lesson I learned when writing my prayers is how the Holy Spirit brings to mind sin that hinders my fellowship with God. Sin in me affects everyone I meet. I have learned that by confessing and turning from my sin, I am immediately restored and able to be used in God's service.

Thanksgiving is a very important part of my prayers. While praise is expressing gratitude for who God *is*, thanksgiving is gratitude to God for what He *does*. If we, as earthly parents, love to hear the words "thank you" from our children, how much more God wants us to thank Him for His blessings. God's greatest blessings do not cost a penny. Money can't buy a glorious sunset or a walk on the beach. Good health is a blessing many people would pay much to attain. God blesses us in hundreds of ways each day. I praise God for who He is and thank Him for what He *does* in my life.

God also has taught me the importance of intercession in my life as a Christian. I believe that the Holy Spirit often breaks loose in others' lives as a discernible result of the prayers of believing Christians. What a joy to see healing and restoration take place in the lives of those we love and know.

Because of what God can do in your life, I recommend that you begin writing your thoughts and prayers. This journal is designed to assist you. My prayer is that God will use this process to help you focus your attention on Him as you pray. God bless you as you begin to fill this spiritual journey.

Carole Lewis
First Place National Director

spiritual

emotional

physical

mental

spiritual

emotional

physical

mental

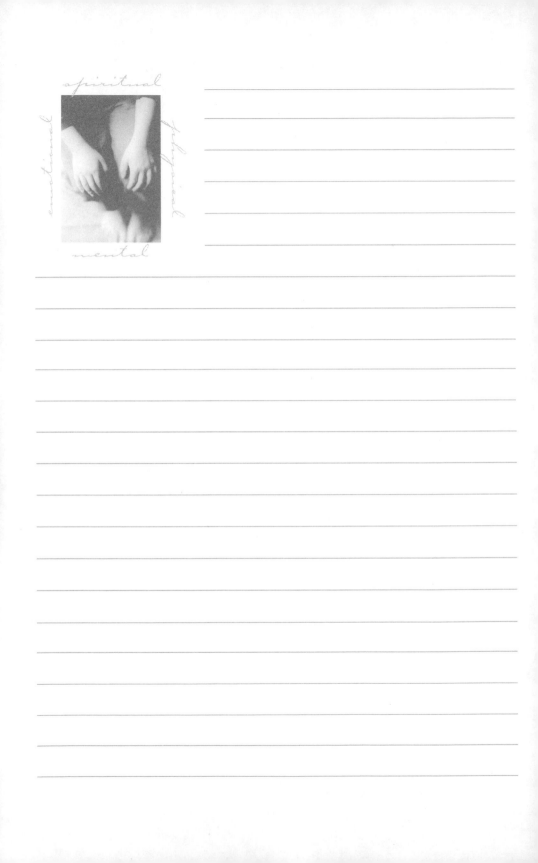

spiritual

emotional

physical

mental

spiritual

emotional

physical

mental

spiritual

emotional

physical

mental

spiritual

emotional

physical

mental

spiritual

emotional

physical

mental

spiritual

emotional

physical

mental

spiritual

emotional

physical

mental

spiritual

emotional   *physical*

mental

spiritual

emotional

physical

mental

spiritual

emotional

physical

mental

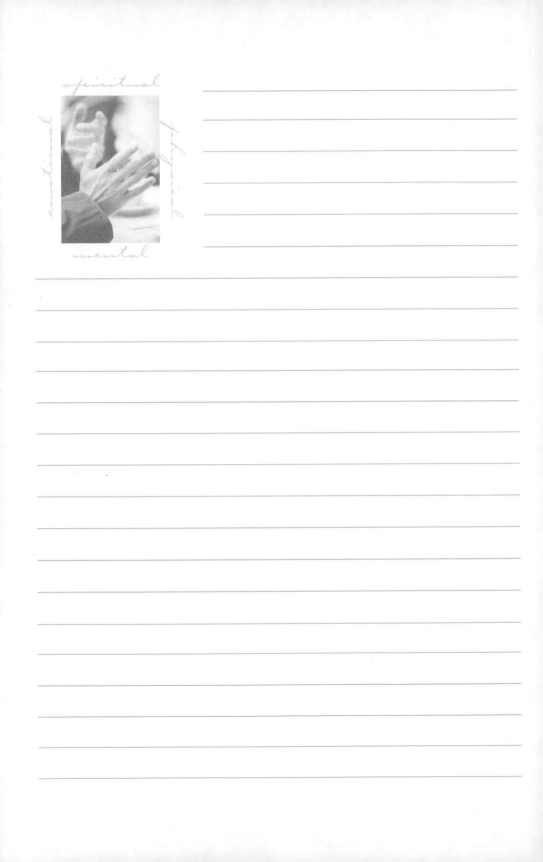

spiritual

emotional

physical

mental

spiritual

emotional

physical

mental

spiritual

emotional

physical

mental

spiritual

emotional

physical

mental

spiritual

emotional

physical

mental

spiritual
emotional
physical
mental

spiritual

physical

emotional

mental

spiritual

emotional

physical

mental

spiritual

emotional　　*physical*

mental

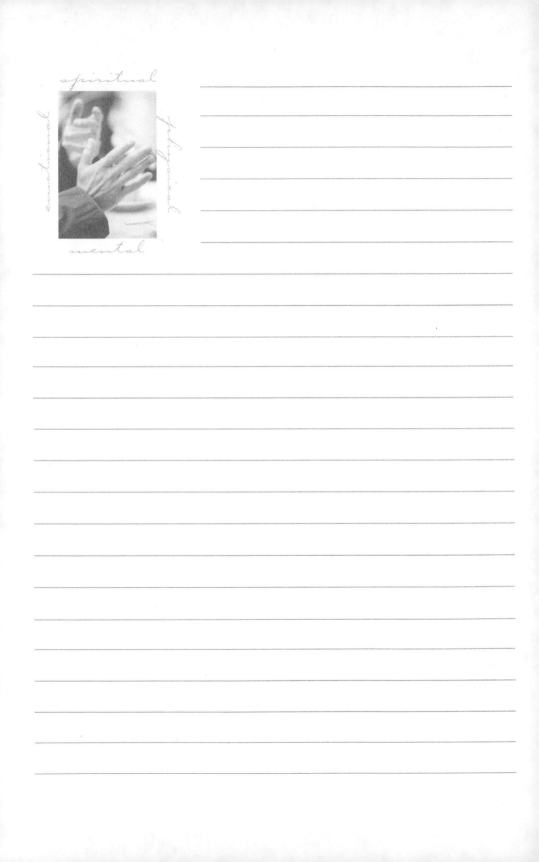

spiritual

emotional

physical

mental

spiritual

emotional

physical

mental

spiritual

emotional

physical

mental

spiritual

emotional

physical

mental

spiritual

emotional

physical

mental

spiritual

emotional

physical

mental

spiritual

emotional

physical

mental

spiritual

emotional

physical

mental

spiritual

emotional

physical

mental

spiritual

emotional

physical

mental

spiritual

emotional

physical

mental

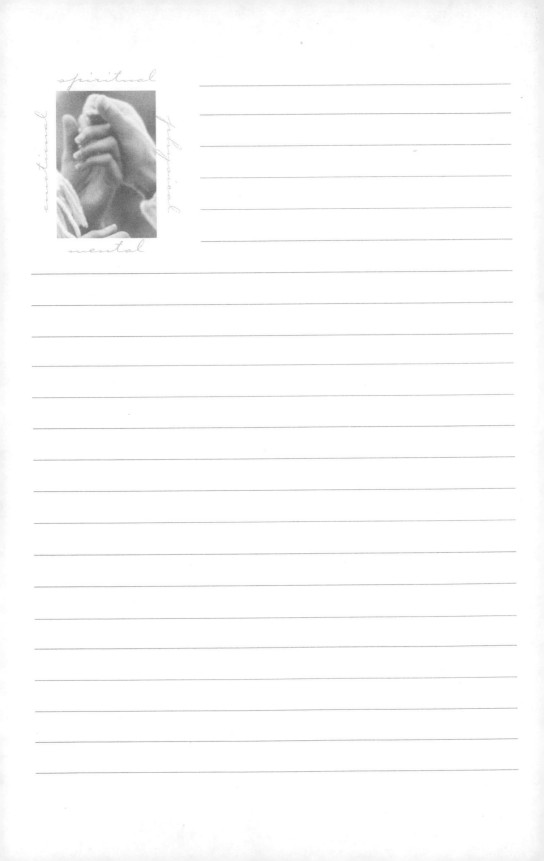

spiritual

emotional

physical

mental

spiritual

emotional

physical

mental

spiritual

emotional

physical

mental

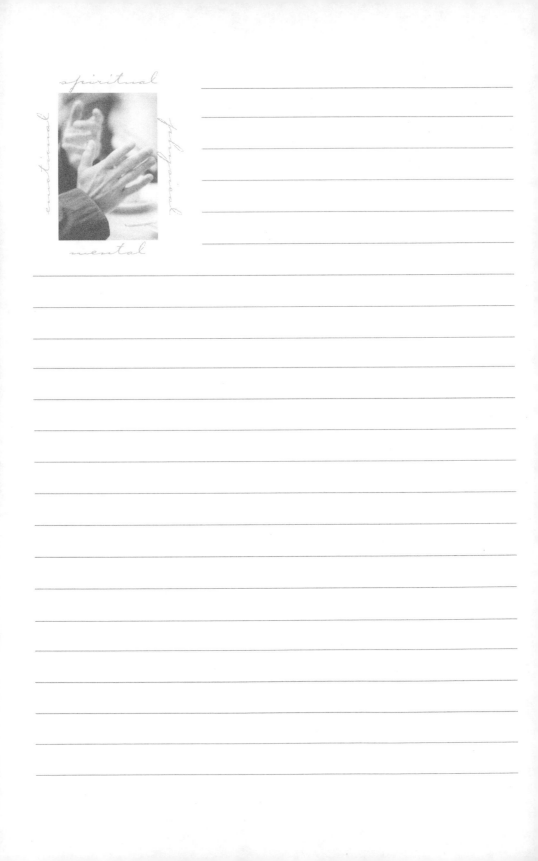

spiritual

emotional

physical

mental

spiritual

emotional

physical

mental

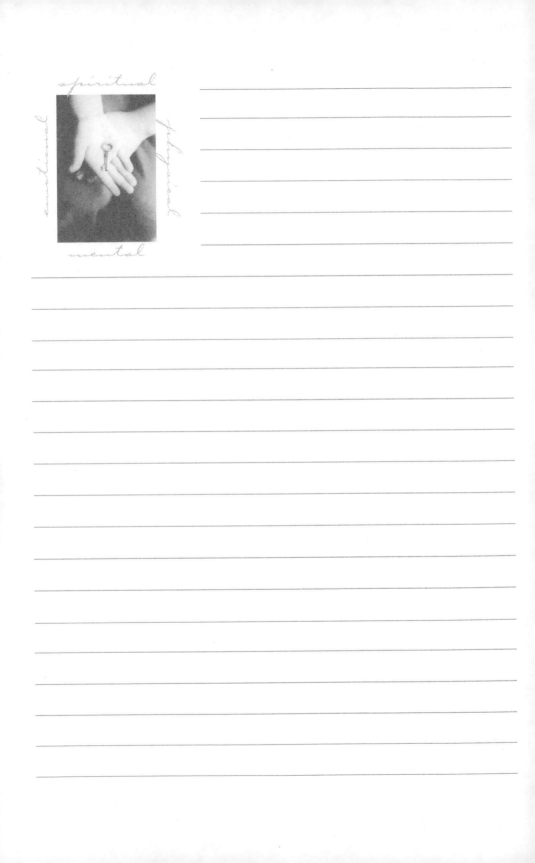

spiritual

emotional

physical

mental

spiritual

physical

emotional

mental

spiritual

emotional

physical

mental

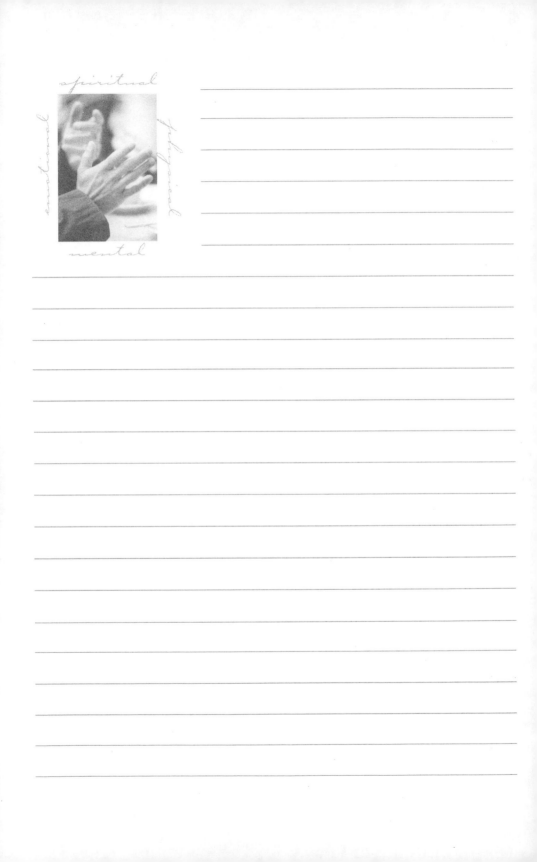

spiritual

emotional physical

mental

spiritual

emotional

physical

mental

spiritual

emotional

physical

mental

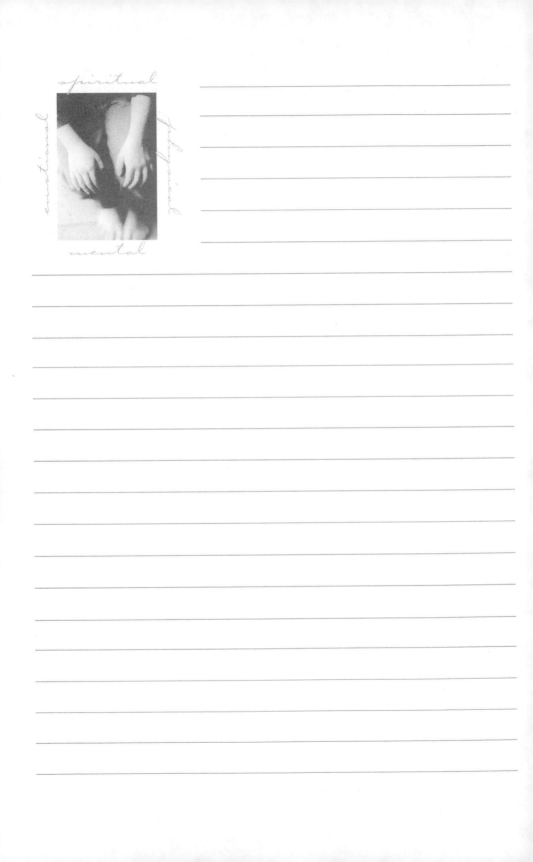

spiritual

emotional

physical

mental

spiritual

emotional

physical

mental

spiritual
emotional
physiological
mental

spiritual

emotional

physical

mental

spiritual

emotional

physical

mental

spiritual

physical

emotional

mental

spiritual

emotional

physical

mental

spiritual

emotional

physical

mental

spiritual

emotional

physical

mental

spiritual

emotional

physical

mental

spiritual

emotional

physical

mental

spiritual

emotional

physical

mental

spiritual

emotional

physical

mental

spiritual

emotional

physical

mental

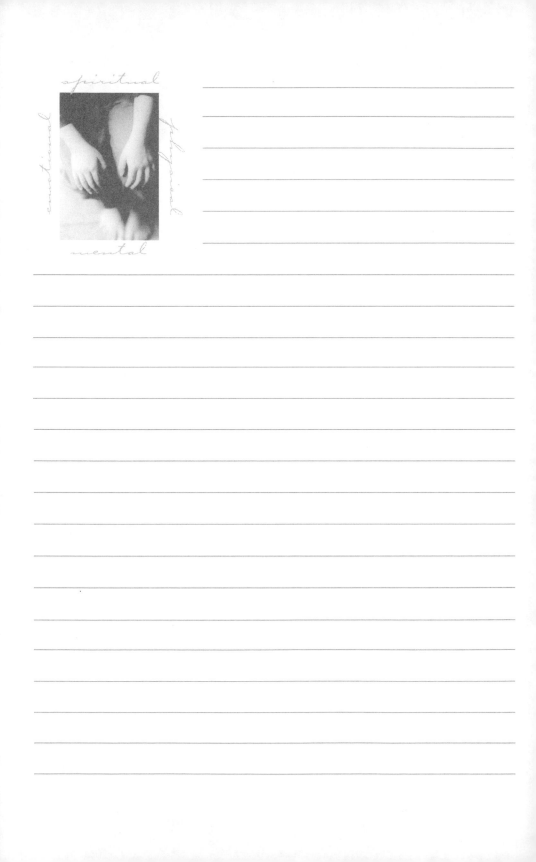

spiritual

emotional

physical

mental

spiritual

emotional

physical

mental

spiritual

emotional

physical

mental

spiritual

emotional

physical

mental

spiritual

emotional

physical

mental

spiritual

emotional

physical

mental

spiritual

emotional

physical

mental

spiritual

emotional

physical

mental

spiritual

emotional

physical

mental

spiritual

emotional

physical

mental

spiritual

emotional

physical

mental

spiritual

emotional

physical

mental

spiritual

emotional

physical

mental

spiritual

emotional

physical

mental

spiritual

emotional

physical

mental

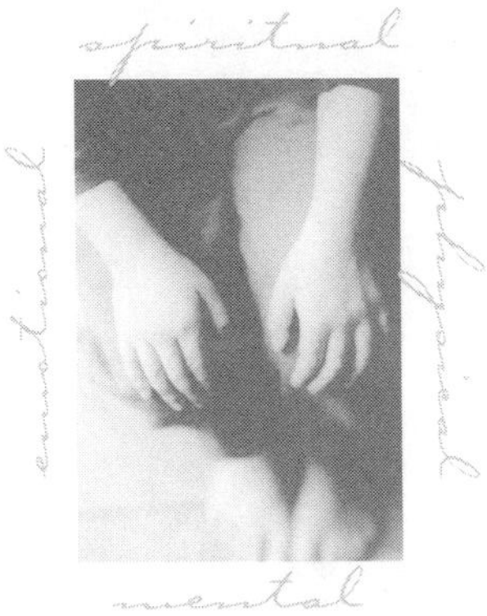
spiritual
physical
mental
emotional

spiritual

emotional

physical

mental

spiritual

emotional

physical

mental

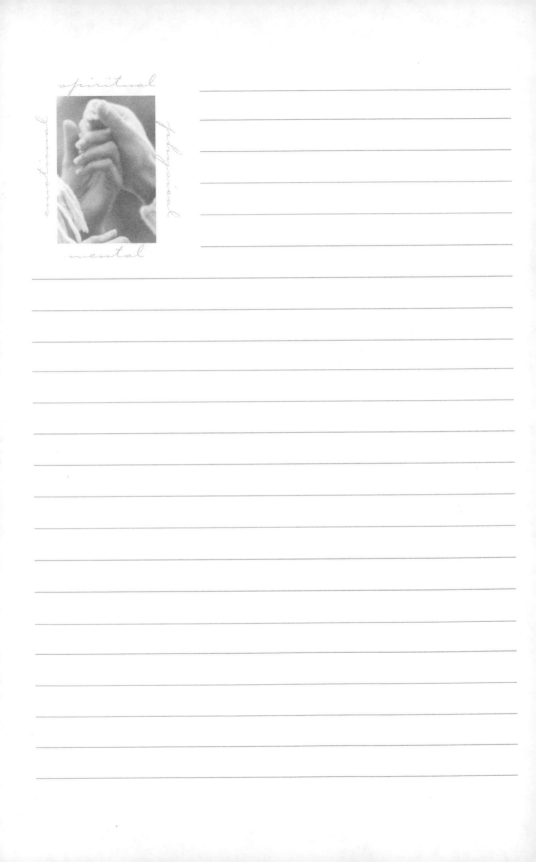

spiritual

emotional

physical

mental

spiritual

emotional

physical

mental

spiritual

emotional

physical

mental

spiritual

emotional

physical

mental

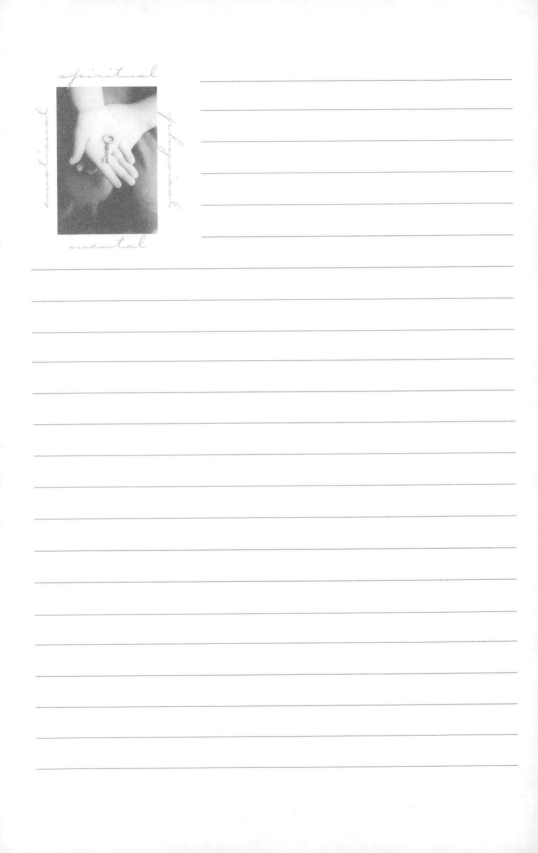

spiritual

emotional

physical

mental

spiritual

emotional

physical

mental

spiritual

emotional

physical

mental

spiritual

emotional

physical

mental

spiritual

emotional

physical

mental

spiritual

emotional

physical

mental

spiritual

emotional

physical

mental

spiritual

emotional

physical

mental

spiritual

emotional

physical

mental

spiritual

emotional

physical

mental

spiritual

emotional

physical

mental

spiritual

emotional

physical

mental